I0419640

A YEAR OF

MAXIMUM

GROWTH

IS GETTING A HAIR TRANSPLANT RIGHT FOR YOU
AND HOW TO GET THE MAXIMUM RESULT

The purpose of this book is to help you decide if a hair transplant procedure is right for you and to help you get the best possible result.

This is a practical handbook that will lead you through all stages of the hair transplanting process: the preparations, the procedure itself and the post-op recovery days and months.

The book explores all aspects of the process in detail, from a patient's perspective.

Some of the things this book will teach you are:

- How F.U.E. hair transplant procedures are executed and what to expect from the moment you step into the clinic. Inside you will find a detailed walk through a Follicular Unit Extraction hair transplanting
- How to handle the inconvenience of the post-surgery hours and days and how to protect the newly transplanted follicles
- How to expedite your recovery and resume your daily routine as quickly as possible.
- And most importantly, how to boost the growth of your newly transplanted hair follicles to a maximum and get the best result possible from your hair transplant procedure.

The book also shares the author's personal experience with F.U.E. hair transplant procedure and provides all the related details, including multiple pictures from the post-surgery ten days and monthly progress for the next 12 months showing all stages of the recovery and growth periods.

Disclaimer

This book is made available for educational purposes only as well as to give you general information and general understanding of the processes and phases related to the hair restoration procedures.

The author of this book is not a licensed physician, and the information contained below should not be used as a substitute for competent medical advice from your surgeon or licensed health professional. Any suggestions, shared observations, and implications reflect the author's personal experience and views. These are the result of years of extensive researching, discussions with certified hair restoration professionals and own experiences. Consult your doctor before following any of the suggestions, ideas, and approaches shared by the author of this book.

Table of Contents

1. INTRODUCTION- THE AUTHOR'S STORY

I started losing my hair in my 20s approximately 15 years ago. I was involved in the fashion industry at that time. Therefore the way I looked was not just of great importance for my self-confidence as an individual but for my professional life as well.

That is why finding a way to combat my hair loss was of crucial importance for me and became a priority number one over the years. I invested years in reading and researching the leading causes of hair loss and the most effective treatments to combat it.

I always stayed on top of all new "cures" for baldness and treatments, claiming not just to stop hair loss, but also completely erase the damages of time and restore its pre-existing condition.

After more than ten years of trying a variety of top-ranked and most recommended products and treatments available on the market, which cost me a small fortune, I decided to finally proceed with an F.U.E. hair transplant procedure in a foreign country overseas.

The hair restoration industry has been rapidly growing over the past years, and the market is oversaturated by a vast variety of hair loss products and treatments, each of which needs to be used for months before any tangible result could be noticed if any at all. Over the years I tried: nutrient-infused hair growth stimulating solutions; a variety of DHT inhibiting shampoos; blood circulation follicle stimulating topical solutions such as Eucapil and Minoxidil (the last being sold under the brand names "Regain" in Europe and "Rogain" here in the United States); a variety of high-end hair stimulating and growth-boosting brand vitamins, and various low-level laser products (laser combs, hats and a handheld devises, etc.).I even signed up for 5-month in-house laser treatment in Phoenix, Arizona, cost me about $5000.

After many years of using hair loss treatments products, I managed to get in control of my progressing hair loss and to slow down the shedding process significantly.

I witnessed many people experiencing pattern hair loss who did not invest the same time, effort and money like myself, losing their hair completely in just a couple to a few years.

Over the years I noticed that some of the products I used worked better than others. I was combining a couple or a few products at the same to time to maximize the effect. I continued to use the ones that I felt worked and gave up on the ones that didn't.

Although I believe that the same products may work differently for each person, in my case, the winning formula for me was the combination of a topical solution (Minoxidil), potent hair vitamins (Anacaps by Ducray) and a hair stimulating and follicle revitalizing shampoo and conditioner Revita, offered by DS Laboratories.

I used many specialized DHT inhibiting topical solutions and shampoos, but I did not see any tangible results on myself. I never used medical Dihydrotestosterone blocking medications, such as Finasteride, due to concerns related to my long term health and well being.
Unfortunately, after attempting many of the available treatments and products available on the market, I never managed to reverse my hair loss and stop it entirely. My hair's condition was slowly but surely getting worse over the years.

The hair transplanting was not an option for me at that time since the surgery (F.U.T) was invasive, leaving a thick, ugly scar on the back of the head. And that combined with the high price tag - around $12-$15 per graft, made the surgical hair restoration out of reach anyway

I reached a point where I had no choice but to start getting into fiber concealers. These helped me cover up my receding hairline until two years later it turned out that I no longer had enough hair for the keratin fibers to hold on to. At that time I had no choice but either finally embrace baldness or have a hair transplant procedure done as a last resort.

Fortunately, the scar-less FUE hair transplant procedures became available a few years later, and the hair restoration clinics started showing significant progress and much better results. Prices dropped significantly (to as low as 50 cents per transplanted follicle after 2016) due to the much higher competition between the clinics.

The new techniques for extracting the follicles and the more advanced technology allowed for much safer procedures and delivery of significantly better results. The progress of the surgical hair restoration also increased the size of the hair restoration procedures making

the transplantation of 5000 grafts in a single session absolutely achievable while that that long ago having 2500 grafts transplanted was considered on the very high end.

Shortly after that advancement, and after months of researching and much consideration, I finally decided to go ahead with a hair transplant procedure. After considering clinics in Mexico, UK, and the US, I decided to have it done in a hair restoration clinic in Istanbul, Turkey in 2017. The strongest influencing factor for me was the recommendation of a close friend of mine who had gone there for his hair restoration and managed to achieve a great result.

I did my best to get myself prepared as well as possible and made sure that I brought everything I thought I would need for my comfort during the first few post-op days and nights.

However, while going over all stages of the entire process, I faced some challenges on the go, I found myself unprepared for.

That is the main reason I decided to share my knowledge and personal experience in this book, hoping it would be of real practical value to you on your journey to optimizing the result of your procedure and avoiding all common threats and mistakes that could negatively impact your desired outcome.

I realized that the best hair restoration clinics and surgeons could only deliver the proper and professional execution of the procedure itself. **However, a big part of the final result is entirely up to you**.

This book emphasizes on your part during the post-op recuperation and growth phases and attempts to provide a "roadmap" that will help you get the most out of your hair transplant procedure with minimum discomfort and disruption of your everyday life.

2. A QUICK GO OVER THE BASICS

2.1. MAIN REASONS FOR ANDROGENIC ALOPECIA (male pattern baldness)

Although a variety of genetic, health and environmental factors may play a role in causing androgenic alopecia in men, it has been determined that the biggest culprit for that permanent type of hair loss in men is due to a hormone (androgen) called Dixydrotestoretone (DHT). Testosterone is metabolized to DHT by the enzyme 5 Alpha-reductase. The AR gene makes the hair follicle receptors that handles the DHT. If your follicle receptors are more sensitive to DHT, they get triggered easily even by small amounts of DHT and as result hair loss occurs more easily. The increased levels of DHT in the hair follicles lead to shorter life cycles of the hairs as well as worsening of the quality of the hair that the hair follicles produce.

2.2. MOST COMMON TYPES OF HAIR LOSS

- **ANDROGENIC ALOPECIA (GENETIC)**
Androgenic Alopecia is a hereditary predisposition, related to increased sensitivity of the hair follicles to increased levels of Dihydrotestosterone due to the 5 alpha-reductase enzyme that is the main reason for converting testosterone into DHT, scientifically proven to be toxic to the hair follicles.

- **ALOPECIA AREATA**

Alopecia Areata is an autoimmune condition where the immune system mistakenly attacks the hair follicles, causing hair to fall off entirely creating round hairless patches in the affected areas.

- **ALOPECIA TOTALIS**

A form of Alopecia Areata, causing a complete loss of scalp hair.

2.3.   MOST COMMON WAYS TO COMBAT HAIR LOSS

- **HAIR TRANSPLANTATION**

F.U.T.-(The "Strip Method")

Hair restoration clinics and surgeons currently rarely use this method. In this method, a strip is harvested from the donor area, and the hairs are manually dissected and implanted in the recipient area (hairline, top or crown).

F.U.E. (Manual Follicular Unit Extraction)

Currently the most popular and widely used methodology for hair transplant procedures in which, the hair follicles are individually harvested from the donor area and manually transplanted onto the recipient area, by a certified hair technician.

Robotic Technique (Follicular Unit Extraction via follicle extraction by a robot)

A version of the Follicular Unit Extraction technique, where a surgeon-controlled robotized medical device is used for performing the follicle extraction and the actual transplanting is done manually by a hair specialist, identical to the FUE procedure.

- ## LOW LEVEL LASER THERAPY

The Food and Drug Administration first approved low-level light therapy in 2007 for the treatment of mild to moderate male pattern hair loss for a laser comb device designed to regrow hair. It has been scientifically proven to have a specific stimulating effect on the hair follicles.

There is a variety of laser therapies and products currently being offered on the marketplace, such as laser hats, laser combs, and laser chairs, Intended to stimulate the hair follicles and increase new hair growth.

- ## CHEMICAL DHT INHIBITORS (Finasteride and Dutasteride)

Finasteride and his brand names Proscar and Propecia, approved by the FDA and scientifically proven to have an antiandrogenic effect, are used primarily in the treatment of enlarged prostate as well as for scalp hair loss.

- ## HAIR GROWTH TOPICAL SOLUTIONS AND SHAMPOOS

Minoxidil
Minoxidil is an antihypertensive vasodilator medication that has been approved by the FDA to treat hair loss and help regrow hair.

It is sold as a liquid solution and foam and offered in two strengths - 2% and 5% topical solution. **Minoxidil** works by helping the blood flow to the **hair** follicles.

Topilutamide

Known more commonly as **Fluridil** and sold under the brand name **Eucapil**, is an anti-androgen medication which is used in the treatment of pattern hair loss in men and women. It is used as a topical medication and applied to the scalp.

Hair growth stimulating shampoos

The high-end hair growth-boosting shampoos usually contain a combination of natural (Organic) ingredients that are strong DHT inhibitors and are clinically proven to lower the level of DHT that gets through into the hair follicles. Some of these shampoo ingredients are: Ketoconazole, Green tea extract, Biotin, Saw Palmetto, Beta-Sitosterol, Pygeum Bark, Gotu Kola, Stinging Nettle Root ,Pygeum Bark, Caffeine, various essential oils such as Pumpkin seed oil, Argan oil, Emu Oil and rosemary oil, Iron, and vitamins B12 & B6.

- **MICRONEEDLING**

  Done by injecting topical PRP (platelet-rich plasma) to help introduce growth factors into the scalp.

- **HAIR LOSS CONCEALERS**

Keratin Fibers

Positively or negatively charged particles, made of keratin from wool, cotton, cellulose or of vegetal origin that bond with the hair thus making it look fuller and thicker.

Hair tattoos (Scalp Micropigmentation)

A type of cosmetic tattoo that imitates hair follicles and creates the illusion of a closely trimmed hair, also used as a visual effect for concealing balding, scars, burns or any skin imperfections.

3. PROS AND CONS OF SURGICAL HAIR RESTORATION

3.1. MAJOR PROS

No pain and visible scarring

Nowadays, hair transplant surgeries are mostly referred to as cosmetic procedures due to the decreased invasiveness and lack of cuts on the scalp.

The times when getting hair transplanted required invasive surgical incisions in the donor area and involved pain and significant healing time are fortunately long gone.

Presently, the hair restoration surgeries have evolved to a stage where the new hair transplanting techniques allow these procedures to be virtually painless, invasive to a minimum and to cause minimum disruption in the patients' lifestyle.

Permanent results

The biggest plus of the hair transplanting is that the effect is considered **permanent.** The transplanted hair follicles are genetically resistant to androgenic alopecia and don't fall off as the rest of the hairs.

Note: Only the newly transplanted follicles are resilient to the toxic impact of **Dihydrotestosterone** (DHT) and are meant to stay. Take into an account that your pre-existing hair follicles will keep getting affected by the DHT, gradually shrinking and producing less and also thinner hairs, which will result in consecutive hair loss.

Provides you with the opportunity to have your hairline redesigned

You will get the chance to participate in the design of your new hairline and shape it up in a different way if that's something you'd like to do. That is up to you, and most surgeons would accommodate their patients' aesthetic vision of how their hairline and final result should look. Try not to be shy and speak up! That would naturally increase the chance of you getting the result you envision.

Creates a natural look

The current techniques in surgical hair restoration have started to provide excellent and natural results, turning the surgical nature of the hair transplanting into a mostly cosmetic procedure.

With the Follicular Unit Extraction technique (F.U.E.), there is no actual incision in the donor area. Each follicle is harvested via miniature punctures instead and relocated over to the hairline, top and crown area, thus aiming at achieving a natural look.

The hair follicles producing one and two strands are placed in the hairline zone and the three and four hair producing follicles, the "density grafts" are transplanted on the top and crown area, thus achieving a completely natural look.

Affordability

Prices have drastically dropped in the past few years, and a hair transplant procedure is presently much more affordable than it was the past.

Many clinics in **Mexico, India, and Turkey** have been exclusively specializing in FUE hair transplanting, annually performing thousands of hair restoration procedures at a reasonable price, as low as up to **50 US cents per hair graft.**

Saves money, time and effort invested in hair loss treatments

The hair transplant procedure is a permanent solution to the hair loss issue. The transplanted hairs are resilient to the toxic impact of DHT and grow the same way as the rest of your hair grows in the donor area, on the back and sides of your head.

The hair transplanting significantly decreases or completely replaces the need for purchasing and using pricey hair growth stimulating medications and DHT inhibitors.

3.2. MAJOR CONS

Requires planning and sufficient time for recovery

The post-surgery recuperation time requires at least a week off work (although surgeons have been claiming otherwise) as well as significant disruption of the usual daily routine.

The recovery process may cause significant inconvenience

Common "side effects" related to the post-op recovery period are: sleep deprivation, affected productivity levels, scalp itching and disruption of the regular lifestyle habits, You will need to adopt and follow particular routines, related to your diet, exercising and also avoid unhealthy habits such as smoking and excessive drinking.

The hair transplant procedures are still quite costly in many countries

The median price per graft in the USA in 2019 is about $6-$7 per graft, which still keeps the hair transplant procedure a luxury venture for many. Fortunately, there are less expensive destinations where the hair restoration procedures are performed at a much more affordable price, such as Turkey, Mexico, and India. The severe competition between the clinics and hair restoration surgeons in these countries have brought the cost per hair graft to as low as 50 cents per hair follicle.

The results take time

The hair transplant procedure is not a "quick fix" and requires time for the results to become noticeable. Although the surgical hair restoration procedure leads to a permanent result, achieving it requires effort and **at least 6-7 months until you can get a visible change of your looks.**

4. THINGS TO CONSIDER BEFORE YOUR PROCEDURE AND WHAT TO EXPECT

Take your time to decide

Maybe you should not rush to a decision on getting a hair transplant procedure done if you are in the early stages of losing your hair.

Keep in mind that the procedure can fix your current level of hair loss, but the rest of your hair will continue to fall out as before.

In case you still decide to get a small scale hair transplant procedure done, be prepared for more surgeries over the years for a full restoration and more permanent results.

Keep in mind, that getting multiple smaller (catch up) procedures would also mean going over the same inconveniences related to the recuperation process and will result in a higher cost per graft due to the smaller scale of each procedure.

On the other hand, technology is continually evolving which leads to lowering the cost per transplanted graft and improved results and effectiveness.

Note: Keep in mind that the keratin fiber concealers can do an excellent job for covering up the bolding areas and help in pushing back the necessity of hair a transplant procedure.

Make sure you have realistic expectations

We are born with an average of 100 000-120 000 hair follicles. Of course, that number varies depending on the person and is also based on race and natural hair color so you should try to set your expectations straight and expect a realistic result.

For example, if you have reached the last stage 7 of pattern baldness on the Hamilton-Norwood scale* you couldn't be expecting to get a full head of hair by having 2000 or 3000 grafts transplanted. That level of hair loss requires around 7000-9000 grafts transplanted to achieve excellent coverage and density

Setting your expectations straight is of extreme importance for your satisfaction from the hair transplant procedure

The result from your hair transplant procedure also depends on the quality of your donor area and not just the number of transplanted grafts

Having a high-density donor area is of vital importance in order to achieve the desired coverage. The level of coverage and hair density does not depend on just the number of transplanted follicles but also on the quality of your donor area and the number of hairs each of your follicles produces. Generally, the hair follicles produce up to four hairs per follicle

The experienced hair surgeons are great at figuring that out and picking the "density" follicles producing 3-4 hairs for the areas on the scalp, necessary for achieving the most volume and the 1-2 hair follicles for outlining your hairline making it look as natural as possible.

* Norwood scale male pattern baldness

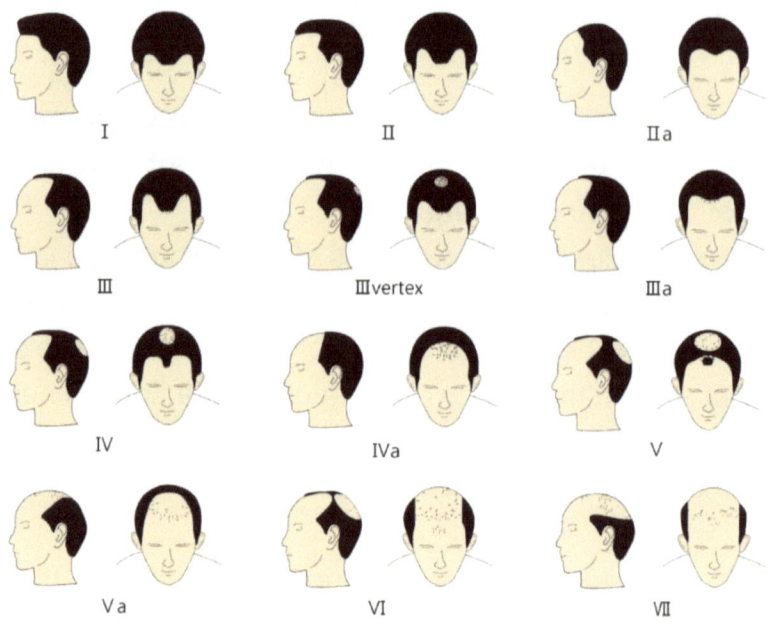

Undergoing the procedure and getting the grafts in is just a beginning

The hair transplant procedure is about 70% of the work, but the rest is up to you so you. To get maximum results you will need to adopt some healthy habits and routines.

Having a certain number of hair follicles immune to DHT transplanted in your balding areas is not good enough to end up having healthy and great looking hair. A large number of side factors also affects the survival rate of your transplanted follicles as well as the looks of your hair in general- your lifestyle, daily routine, diet, stress levels, exercising habits, general health condition, etc.

You should also take into account that the newly transplanted follicles are more vulnerable and require special care and attention. Adopting some healthy habits will result in improving the general quality of your blood, which provides the "food" for your hair follicles, and would most certainly get you closer to the desired result.

Ensure enough time for post-op recovery

It is highly recommended that you avoid traveling a long distance and fully relax the first few days after the surgery.

Traveling long distance may increase the risk of a negative impact on your post-surgery recuperation process It will increase the chances for contaminating and infecting the transplanted area which is extremely sensitive in the first 24-72 hours post-op

Plan your accommodation ahead of time

Unfortunately while selling their services and competing for patients, most hair restoration clinics and surgeons diminish the significance of the post-surgery 48-72 hour period. You should have in mind that the first 72 hours after the procedure are critical and are of vital importance for your final result. It is best that you do your best to free up at least 2-3 days after your procedure and avoid long distance traveling so you can take your time and rest.

It is also claimed by many hair restoration surgeons that long distance traveling is possible on the very next day after the procedure and that the patients could resume their usual and business daily routine in about 2 or 3 days post-op. I find that a bit too optimistic. Do yourself a favor and consider staying at your hotel room and try to put aside your work responsibilities for at least 3-4 days after the surgery.

The procedure itself and the post-op healing process may be painless for most patients but are not as nondisruptive as most clinics, and hair surgeons make it look.

Prepare yourselves for hardly getting any sleep the first night

You shouldn't expect to sleep much on the first night after the procedure. Being told that you could harm or entirely ruin your result by your surgeon would most likely prevent you from getting a good night sleep in the first two or 3 days.

In case you have any important engagements such as family matters or business duties or anything that requires you being at a 100%, do your best to push these back for at least four or five days after the procedure.

Expect your hair to be trimmed close to the skin if you are in for more than 2000 grafts

Cutting your hair very short will provide your surgeon with direct and easy access to your hair follicles in the donor area for quicker and more precise extraction and will also help the transplanting onto the recipient area. Most surgeons would mention that ahead of time, but it is good to expect that happening and get yourself mentally prepared regardless.

Do not expect any dramatic progress for at least five or six months after the procedure

Keep in mind that most likely you won't be able to see significant results for at least a 5-6 months after the surgery. The hair transplant procedure may be a permanent solution but is not a "quick fix" So if let's say your wedding day is two months away, do yourself a favor and don't expect that you will get a full head of hair in just two months.

Your transplanted hairs will temporarily fall out due to "shock loss" before starting to produce new hairs.

The human hairs have their natural life cycles (anagen, catagen, and telogen) and life longevity between two and seven years. Know that extracting the hair follicles from their natural habitat (the donor area) for repositioning will put them in a state of distress. The vast majority of them gets into a dormant mode. Before to start producing new hairs, most hair follicles push out the existing hairs. Your existing hairs falling off means that the follicles are resetting and clearing out the way for the new hairs and new growth.

Many hair restoration patients get distressed when the "shock loss" occurs, especially being able to see themselves with more visible hairs right after the transplant procedure before losing most of them within three weeks post-op.

The good news is that not all follicles participate in the "Shock Loss" stage. Some of them manage to maintain their current growth and life cycle and don't fall out.

Although the number of hairs you will lose due to the shock loss is strictly subjective, you should be expecting to lose up to

80% of your newly transplanted hairs between the 2nd and the 8th-week post-surgery. That is fine and a part of the recovery process. What is of importance are the newly transplanted hair follicles that shortly after the "shock loss" stage get back to work and start producing new hairs.

5. A WALK THROUGH THE FUE HAIR TRANSPLANT PROCEDURE

5.1. PRELIMINARY CONVERSATION WITH YOUR SURGEON

You will most likely have a discussion with your surgeon before your transplant procedure as a final go over the details. Now is the time to speak out and make your surgeon aware of what exactly you are hoping to achieve- density, graft location, the shape of your hairline, etc.

Speaking out at this point is your last chance to make sure that there is no miscommunication and everything will be done according to your previous conversations, before your actual hair transplant procedure.

5.2. GETTING YOUR HAIRLINE DESIGNED (in case that is a part of what you are in for)

Some surgeons do it themselves during the pre-op conversation, and some have a designated hairline designer that will go over how you envision your new hairline shape and will design your hairline accordingly with a medical marker.

5.3.   PRE-PROCEDURE PREPARATIONS

That's when in most cases you will be asked to undress and put on a hospital shirt or gown (usually provided by the clinic), and have your hair trimmed close to the skin (in most cases via hair-clippers). After that is done, you will be placed on the surgical table, face down, for the follicle extraction.

5.4.   THE ANESTHETIC STAGE

Your surgeon will start injecting the anesthetic shots in your donor area. You will be able to feel the first two or three punctures before your head goes numb in the donor area and you lose sensation completely.

Try not to stress out before your procedure. It is supposed to be completely painless aside from the first few anesthetic shots. Once the unpleasant sensation from getting the first few shots is gone, you won't be able to feel anything. Just try to relax and let the professionals do their job.

5.5.   FOLLICLE EXTRACTION

The first stage of the transplant procedure is the extraction of the hair follicles. That is when each follicle will be extracted individually, placed on a sterilized gauze pad and kept in a sanitary environment for the next stage of the hair transplant procedure, which is the actual transplanting of the extracted follicles.

The follicle extraction shouldn't take more than 1.5-2 hours, depending on the number of follicles harvested and the number of technicians/surgeons performing the procedure.

Lunch break (for full head procedures, over 2500 grafts)

Most clinics and surgeons strive to maximize the comfort of their patients by providing a 30-40 minute lunch break between the extraction and the transplant part of the procedure.

5.6.   PREPARING THE RECIPIENT AREA

Your hair surgeon will ask you to turn around, usually in a semi-seated position (usually a 45-degree angle) for the pinhole punctures that are typically made with a thin, custom-made surgical blade. Of course, after the anesthetic shots are injected so the recipient area becomes completely numb and there is no sensation in the transplant area whatsoever.

5.7.   TRANSPLANTING THE HAIR FOLLICLES

At this stage, the already extracted hair follicles will be getting inserted in the newly punctured pinholes in your recipient area. Often for larger scope procedures (over 2500-3000 grafts), there is more than one technician involved. In my case there were 2 of them, working simultaneously.

Since the time required for the entire procedure can be significant, many clinics provide some form of entertainment for their patients, like watching a movie or listening to some music.

5.8.   BANDAGE PLACEMENT

Your surgeon will place a bandage on your donor to keep it sterile and prevent infection.

After the procedure is finally done, you will be asked to stand up and go to the dressing room where you will need to change.
It is essential that you bring a button down shirt or top with a zipper, so you don't have to risk anything touching or rubbing against your transplanted area.

6. POST SURGERY RECOVERY STAGES AND WHAT TO EXPECT AFTER THE PROCEDURE

Once the procedure is completed and you get dressed, you will most likely be dropped off back at your hotel.

The reputable hair restoration clinics usually provide post-surgery transportation and complimentary hotel accommodation for a day or two. It is of great importance that you have the ride back arranged in advance, in case that is not provided by the clinic

6.1. THE FIRST 24HOIRS AFTER THE PROCEDURE

Your surgeon will most likely advise you to be careful not to bump or touch your transplanted area under any circumstances since you could easily pull out the transplanted follicles and ruin your result.

That is usually when most transplant patients begin to realize that not everything depends on their surgeon and they will have to do their part to protect their result. Many hair restoration patients end up being unprepared and find themselves feeling uncomfortable once they leave the clinic.

Unfortunately, most hair restoration clinics do not provide particular post-op products that could protect their patients' transplanted area so it would be entirely up to you if and how good you'll safeguard your newly transplanted follicles.

Keep in mind that the newly transplanted follicles are planted loosely in the recently punctured pinholes on your scalp and are extremely easy to pull out just by touching them.

The first 24 hours are critical until the pinholes start gradually shrinking and tightening up.

Realistically you should not be expecting to get any sleep at all the first night post-op, maybe the second one as well.

6.2. THE FIRST NIGHT AFTER THE PROCEDURE

As mentioned above, safeguarding the transplanted area the first night after the procedure is of vital importance so you will have a few options :

- To postpone going to bed and stay awake for a while. That ensures more time for the pinholes in your recipient area to start shrinking and prevents the chance of unconsciously touching it in your sleep or rubbing it against the pillow.

- Go to bed for a few hours and use a special orthopedic pillow that supports your neck, elevates your head and prevents you from turning in your sleep and moving your head*.

- It is still possible for you to start scratching and touching your head in your sleep, so you should think of a way to restrain your hands in some way to limit their reach to the transplanted area.

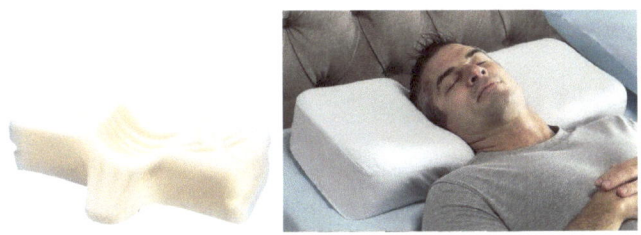

- To try to get some sleep in a semi-seated position. Many transplant patients do that and use a travel neck pillow.

6.3.   DAY ONE POST-SURGERY - bandage removal

The first day is the most critical. The newly transplanted hair follicles are still extremely vulnerable even a gentle touching .of the transplanted area may have a very negative impact on your result down the road.

Do not forget that the pinholes on your scalp are still in the process of shrinking, and any direct contact with the recipient area can lead to pulling out the newly inserted follicles.

It is strongly recommended that you do your best to avoid traveling the next day The best you can do is to try to safeguard the recipient area, and the best way of doing that is to avoid moving around too much and engaging in too many daily activities.

Your head bandage will most likely be removed the next day after your procedure.

Taking off the bandage is a routine procedure that requires just a few moments and is completely painless.

6.4.   WEEK ONE POST-SURGERY

Please, do not forget that the first 7-8 days after the procedure are of vital importance for your final result.

Below is an overview of what to expect and how to handle it.

- **Light head swelling**

Please note, that swelling (regardless of the anti-inflammatory medications) is very common, and the scale is strictly individual. Almost everyone gets light to medium head swelling, usually within 2-3 days after the procedure.

The best you can do is to keep taking anti-inflammatory medications and elevate your head while sleeping. Try not to panic and accept it as a part of the process! It usually takes 2-5 days for the swelling to go away.

- **Scabs forming and scalp dryness**

Know that little crusts will start forming in the affected areas on your scalp a couple of days after your transplant procedure.

You should keep in mind that the scabs are a part of your skin's natural healing process and appear as an expected result from the multiple pinholes you will get during the procedure.

How to remove the scabs

The proper way to remove the crusts is to be patient and do it slowly and gradually, by softening up the epidermal layer **on your head. That could be done by using a mist spray to moisturize the skin on your head and also by using medical skin softening lotion before washing**. The right way to do that is to apply a thin layer of the moisturizer on your head with gentle tapping moves and to keep it sit for a couple of minutes before washing your head (not before the 3rd day after the procedure).

Generally, it takes seven to ten days for the scabs to soften up and fall off completely

IMPORTANT NOTE: Attempting to remove the crusts from your head forcefully could easily result in pulling out the transplanted follicles that are right underneath. It is imperative that you don't try to expedite the process.

6.5.   WEEK 1-3 AFTER THE PROCEDURE

After you have successfully gotten through the critical first week, you will most likely start noticing the following:

- **Scabs are starting to fall off or have fallen off completely.**

- **There is noticeable redness in the recipient/transplanted areas.**

    That is absolutely normal. Although that's strictly individual, usually the redness starts fading away 7 to 14 days after the procedure.

- **Healing of the donor area**

    The **donor area** on the back of your head should have entirely healed by the end of the first week.

- **Scalp numbness**

    It is normal to still feel some numbness on your scalp during the first 3-4 weeks after the procedure, sometimes even longer. After the numbness goes away, it will most likely be replaced by a light tingling sensation and itching. That is normal and is a part of the healing process.

- **Immediate hair growth**

    Many of you may even be able to notice fast hair growth of the already transplanted hairs.

6.6.   1-2 MONTHS AFTER THE PROCEDURE (Shock loss & Dormant stage)

Welcome to the "shock loss" stage!
During that period your transplanted hair will start falling out. Be aware that losing most of the newly transplanted hairs due to " shock loss" is normal. That is a part of the process and has nothing to do with the success of your hair restoration procedure.

Unless you know what to expect, this stage could cause a lot of distress for many hair transplant patients.

- **A quick explanation of the "shock loss" process**

During this period, the already transplanted follicles release the old hairs in order to "restart" themselves while adapting to the new environment. Many of the newly transplanted follicles become dormant before starting to produce new healthy hairs.

So be prepared for the " shock loss" and get excited rather than stressed out.

Only a certain percentage of the transplanted follicles will undergo that phase, and that number is strictly individual. It is essential for you to remember that what is not visible at that moment is that the hair transplant procedure is all about and that's the newly transplanted, "healthy" hair follicles.

Note: The " shock loss" may affect between 30% and 80% of the transplanted follicles.

It is important not to think that your procedure was unsuccessful during that phase and try to stay positive.

6.7. 3-4 MONTHS AFTER THE PROCEDURE (the new growth stage)

After the first couple of months, your transplanted follicles will slowly start getting out of the dormant phase and begin producing new hairs.

The newly growing hairs will look thinner and with less density in the beginning. The human's hair follicles usually produce between one and four hairs each. However, at the beginning of the growing phase, there will be one hair coming out of each follicle at a time until all hairs grow out of each follicle as genetically predetermined.

During this stage, the best you could do to accelerate the newly transplanted hairs growth is to maintain a healthy daily routine- exercising regularly, sleeping at least 7 hours a day and following a highly nutritious diet.

Note, that it is strictly individual when exactly you'd be getting into the growing phase. Sometimes it starts on the 2nd month after the transplant procedure, sometimes it may take a little longer. Keep in mind that whether you will start getting new hair growth on early stages or not, that has nothing to do with the result you will end up with. Some "slow growers" end up having better results than some " early birds."

6.8. 6-8 MONTHS AFTER THE PROCEDURE (Accelerated Growth Phase)

This is probably the most exciting phase. The transplanted follicles start producing more and fuller hairs. At this stage, you will most likely be able to see most of the hairs already out and thickening up. During this period, most people start noticing a drastic change in the look of their hair and begin to feel already happy with their results.

Note: Depending on the individual, some get in that stage with a slight delay, between the 8th or 9th month after the hair transplant procedure.

6.9.   9-12 MONTHS AFTER THE PROCEDURE (Continuous growth and hair thickening)

About 80% -90% of your hairs should already be out and already thickened, nicely blending with the rest of your hair.

6.10.   12-14 MONTHS AFTER THE PROCEDURE – The final result

Your new hair growth is 100% completed so at this stage you will be able to see the full result from your surgery.

Most hair transplant patients need up to 12 months for a complete re-growth but some "slow growers" may need an extra couple of months to achieve or even surpass the same result.

7. HAIR GROWTH TIME FRAMES

After all of you transplanted follicles reach the maximum of their genetically predetermined potential (usually between 1 and four hairs per hair follicle), they will start going through the same natural life stages as the rest of your hair. So in the future, you will be experiencing the same natural hair shedding cycles but also new revolving hair growth.

0-2 months - 20%
2-4 months - 40%
4-8 months- 80% *
8-12 months- 90 % *
12-14 months- 100% *

*Note: Please, keep in mind that the above time frames and percentages are general and may vary, depending on the person. Some hair transplant patients may need more time to get out of the "shock loss" stage but catch up during the "growth" stage and end up with the same phenomenal result.

8. HOW TO PREPARE FOR YOUR PROCEDURE (DO'S AND DON'TS)

8.1. DO'S

Get yourself well prepared

Try to bring everything you will need after the procedure. The reputable clinics that strive for their patients' ultimate satisfaction and quality of service usually provide everything necessary in terms of aftercare so that the post-op hours are as less disruptive and comfortable as possible.

A part of the items the hair restoration clinics usually provide are painkillers, anti-inflammatory medication, softening conditioner that will be helping you get off the little crusts that will form in the transplant area where the new grafts were placed, neutral PH shampoos, and antibiotics. However, before you get in for your procedure, it is good to ask what precisely the clinic is going to be providing you with. Make sure that you will get everything necessary with you.

Many most reputable clinics even go the extra mile and provide accommodation included in the price of the procedure.

It is vital that you ensure your rest after the procedure and especially during the first night.

You will have to be very careful and avoid touching and rubbing your head at any cost!

Make sure that you bring a suitable pillow that will elevate your head and support your neck in the first few nights after your procedure. A special orthopedic pillow will help you avoid excessive head swelling and will decrease the chances for rubbing the recipient area and risk pulling out the transplanted hair follicles. Also, bring a **button down shirt or a top with a zipper** which you can put on right after the procedure without risking to touch the recipient area while changing your clothes.

Boost your immune system and detoxify your body

The quality of your blood is of great importance for the post-op stages as well as the speed your new hairs will start growing with, their thickness and look. If your blood is in a good state, that would most likely positively affect the result from your hair transplant procedure. Having pure, oxygenated, healthy blood could help you boost your new hair growth, accelerate your recuperation period and also likely diminish the scale of the " shock loss" stage.

Get a good night sleep the night before the procedure

It is possible that you won't be able to sleep much after the procedure so try to go to bed early the night before. It would be fantastic if you could steal a couple of hours of sleep during the surgery itself. That would be possible since you won't be feeling any pain whatsoever.

Figure out a way to protect the sensitive are after the procedure

Unfortunately not much is available on the market to help during the first few days after the procedure so you may need to get creative. Even the most reputable clinics don't offer any specialized products that can be of real help during the first post-op days and nights. From this point on, safeguarding the newly transplanted hair follicles will be entirely your responsibility. The least you can do is to use a special orthopedic pillow while you sleep, a suitable hat when going outdoors, and keep your hands off your head.

Make sure you are taking the post-op medications prescribed by your surgeon

Most clinics usually provide anti-inflammatory pills, corticosteroids, and antibiotics. They will neutralize the post-op physical discomfort or ache, decrease the inflammation and prevent your head from infection.

Also, use the aftercare products, recommended or provided by your surgeon. Often the clinics provide a particular kind of skin softening lotion and a 5.5PH medical shampoo.

In case the aftercare products are not provided by the clinic, make sure that you bring your own.

Wash your head gently and with extreme caution

You must wait until the pinholes on your head close off completely, which will take about 48 hours after the procedure. You should start washing your head on the third day after your surgery. The safest way to do that is by using a very soft sponge for applying the softening lotion and the shampoo on your head. Pour a few drops of the shampoo on the sponge and hold it under lukewarm water until it gets foamy. Start applying the foam on your head in both the donor and recipient area very gently and with vertical tapping moves. **DO NOT RUB OR PRESS!**

Wash the foam away by just holding your head under a low-pressure spray of lukewarm water, at least 1-1.5 feet (40-50 centimeters) away from the shower head. Avoid washing your head with cold or hot water since that could harm the newly transplanted follicles.

Many surgeons recommend the use of medical skin softening lotion before washing, to prevent excessive dryness of the scalp and help to soften up the crusts that start forming a few days after the procedure.

The way to apply the lotion is the same described above- via a soft sponge and with gentle tapping moves. Let it sit on your head for a couple of minutes and then proceed with the washing.

CAUTION! Do not use your fingertips to apply the lotion or the shampoo on your scalp in the first week after the surgery! That could lead to pulling out some of the transplanted follicles.

Eat more nutritious foods

The human hairs are made of protein, named Keratin. To boost your hair's growth, it is strongly recommended that you increase the protein intake by at least 30% during the growth post-surgery months, ideally to about 2 grams per kilo (2 lbs) of body weight (or 1 gram per pound).

Making sure that your diet is rich in nutrients-proteins, essential fatty acids, fibers, vitamins (b6 and b12) and minerals, is of importance for your hair and especially for the newly transplanted follicles. They will need plenty of nutrients to quickly go through the recovery stages and subsequently start producing new healthy hairs.

Keep yourself hydrated

Drinking a lot of water will cleanse your body and help to detoxify your blood while increasing the oxygen levels in your blood cells, hence the amount of oxygen supply to the hair follicles. That is of great importance for your newly transplanted hair grafts and their growth.

Exercise regularly

Regular exercising is strongly recommended after the first two weeks from your procedure. The light to moderate physical activities* help to increase the blood circulation to the transplanted area. That ensures access of sufficient amount of oxygen and nutrients to your hair follicles.

*Important note:
Avoid any physical activity during the first post-surgery week and high-intensity workouts for at least 3-4 weeks after your procedure. If you don't, you would be risking your hair follicles to get pushed out due to the increased blood pressure.

Rest as much as possible
Try getting as much sleep as you can during the post-op recovery period.

Sleep helps restore, revitalize and regenerate the brain and the cells in our bodies. Make sure you get enough good night sleep, so you accelerate the healing process.

8.2. DON'TS

Do not touch, rub or scratch the recipient area
As mentioned earlier, doing that will inevitably result in hurting or pulling out some of the newly transplanted hair follicles. You may even want to clip your fingernails deep to decrease the chances of accidentally damaging or removing the newly transplanted hair follicles.

Do not smoke
Smoking brings the blood pressure down and decreases the blood circulation through the vessels that ensure the supply of necessary nutrients and oxygen for your hair follicles when they are most vulnerable.

If you are a smoker, do your best to not smoke at all for at least one week after the procedure. In case that would be too difficult to achieve, try to limit smoking to the bare minimum and avoid inhaling the smoke.

Do not drink any alcohol

Do your best not to drink any alcoholic beverages for at least one week after your hair transplant procedure. Alcohol acts as a blood thinner and will negatively impact the quality of the blood that goes to the transplanted hair follicles.

Also note, that mixing up the anti-inflammatory medication and painkillers with alcohol of any kind is not a good idea.

Do not wash your head In the first two days post-op

As mentioned earlier, it is of crucial importance that you don't wash your head until after two days after the surgery, so you don't pull out any of the transplanted grafts.

However, It is mandatory that you start gently washing your head from the 3rd day onwards, so you maintain the transplanted area clean and avoid bacterial infection.

Washing your head once a day will also help you remove the crusts easier.

NOTE: Make sure you follow the washing instructions in the Do's section.

Do not put any chemical containing products on your scalp

Most hair styling or coloring products (hairsprays, gels, hair dyes, etc.) contain aggressive chemicals that can negatively impact your hair follicles and may worsen or significantly harm your final result.

Avoid heavy lifting and excessive physical activities

As mentioned in the Do's section, light aerobic exercising is even strongly recommended two weeks after the procedure. However, extreme physical activity, heavy lifting, and high-intensity workouts must be avoided for at least a few weeks after the procedure. That will create excess blood pressure and can harm the transplanted follicles.

Do not touch or try to pull out your scabs

As mentioned in section 5.4. above, touching and trying to forcefully remove the crusts from your donor and the transplanted area is a major Don't since that can result in pulling out some of the newly transplanted follicles.

You must be patient and wait until the crusts gradually start falling off by themselves, usually 7-10 days after they appear.

Avoid direct sun exposure and extreme temperatures

After the hair transplant procedure, the affected areas will be overly sensitive to any extreme sensations and temperatures. That is one of the reasons to choose a season for your procedure, when the temperature is neither too high, nor too low.

9. CHOOSING THE RIGHT CLINIC

9.1. DO YOUR RESEARCH ON THE CLINIC/SURGEON

Doing your due diligence and checking out the clinics and surgeons you have shortlisted is of vital importance. Many hair transplant patients make a common mistake and often lured by the price neglect to address other facts about the clinics. Generally the internet is quite a good and informative source as it comes to researching hair transplantation clinics.

- **Check the clinic's or surgeon's certifications, licenses and insurance**

You may want to know if your surgeon is a really certified hair transplant physician and not just a hobby technician. In case you don't find the clinic's certificates and proof of insurance on the clinic's website, do not hesitate to reach out directly to the clinic and request that information to be provided directly to you.

- **Find out more about the reputation of the clinics you are considering**

Generally the internet hair restoration forums are a good source for such information. Remember that aside from your time and money, you will also be trusting the clinic or surgeon you choose with the follicles in your donor area. Look up past patients' experiences with the same clinic or surgeon.

Most reputable clinics and surgeons usually get plenty of reviews online so try to read the online reviews before making the first contact with the clinics you shortlisted.

It is always good to get at least a few unbiased opinions from former patients. The hair forums and independent personal blogs are generally an excellent source of unbiased information on hair transplant clinics.

Of course, having a personal recommendation from someone you know and trust is the best case scenario so you can also ask around for any suggestions.

- **Look for someone you know personally for recommendation**

There is nothing better than getting a recommendation by someone you know personally.

10. FIRST CONTACT WITH THE CLINIC AND MAIN QUESTIONS TO ASK

The vast majority of the people considering hair transplant procedure usually do not know where to begin and what exactly to do when deciding on which clinic they should put their trust in and what kind of questions they should ask.

Asking the right questions is of great importance for getting a positive outcome from your hair transplant procedure.

Below is a list of the most important things to do and questions you should ask the clinics you have shortlisted, before deciding which one to trust.

10.1. MAKE SURE YOU ARE ON THE SAME PAGE WITH YOUR SURGEON

When you get in contact with the clinics you are targeting, be clear about what result you want to achieve. Discuss the desired outcome and the scope of the procedure ahead of time. Having a very clear picture in your head of what you want to achieve is of vital importance for getting the desired result at the end.

Don't be shy and share your full expectations with your surgeon - the coverage and density you are hoping to achieve, hairline shape, etc.

It is always good to provide photos and any visual representation of the result you are hoping for. That will diminish the chance for any misunderstanding with your surgeon.

Discuss how many transplanted hair follicles will be necessary to get the coverage and density you are hoping for and whether that can be achieved in a single procedure.

Many hair transplant patients walk away disappointed because they did not speak out and share their expectations before the procedure. Try not to be one of them!

10.2. WHAT TECHNIQUE WILL BE USED FOR THE FOLLICLE EXTRACTION

You want to make sure you will be getting a Follicular Unit Extraction procedure and not the invasive surgical FUT procedure where an incision is made in the donor area on the back and sides of the head.

It will not do any harm to get reassurance by your surgeon on the method they will use for harvesting the follicles from the donor area.

The FUT (strip) method is considered obsolete in the countries where the hair restoration industry is in line with the current standards.

10.3. ARE THE TRANSPORTATION AND HOTEL ACCOMMODATION PROVIDED BY THE CLINIC

I am sure you don't want to find yourself in a position of having to deal with finding transportation by yourself back to your hotel, right after the surgery. That's why it is best to make sure that you have that covered ahead of time.

The reputable clinics provide complementary hotel accommodation for up to 3 nights and ground transportation between the airport, the hotel, and the clinic, free of charge.

10.4. ARE ALL NECESSARY POST-OP MEDICATIONS PROVIDED BY THE CLINIC

The post-op medications and things you would most likely need, include: anti-inflammatory drugs, painkillers, corticosteroids, 5.5 PH shampoo, softening lotion (for removing the scabs), special orthopedic pillow or a travel neck pillow, something to guard your transplanted area with, special post-procedure travel hat...etc.).

Most reputable hair restoration clinics provide all post-surgery medications that neutralize completely any painful sensation you may get after the procedure, chances for swelling or physical discomfort that you may feel after the procedure.

11. THE AUTHOR'S HAIR TRANSPLANT PROCEDURE

11.1. PRE-SURGERY PREPARATIONS

Below are some of the things I did to enhance my results and get the maximum out of my hair transplant procedure.

- I went through a 2-week herbal detox program before my procedure.

- Continuously took vitamins to boost my hair growth. I went with ANACAPS by Ducray.

- Increased my weekly exercising to 45-60 min, 3-4 times a week. (3 weeks after the procedure)

- I did increase my protein intake by 30% to 2-2.5 grams per kilogram (2 Lbs) of my body weight.

- I started using a hair growth-boosting shampoo (Revita) and hair conditioner from DS Laboratories, a US brand specializing in advanced innovative high-end hair products.

- I discontinued the use of any hair styling products and mainstream shampoos* for at least ten months after the procedure.

    *due to the chemicals that are many manufacturers use in the making

11.2. ITEMS I TOOK WITH ME ON MY TRIP TO THE CLINIC

- A custom made post-op pillow
- A custom made sterile fedora hat. I used the fedora hat since it seemed much safer for my transplanted area.
- A few comfortable full zipper sweaters.

11.3. MEDICATIONS AND ITEMS PROVIDED BY THE CLINIC

- **Painkillers**
- **Corticosteroids**- considered the most effective anti-inflammatory medication
- **Antibiotics** which I took for three days after the procedure
- **5.5 PH Medical grade shampoo**
- **Skin softening lotion** for softening up and removing the scabs

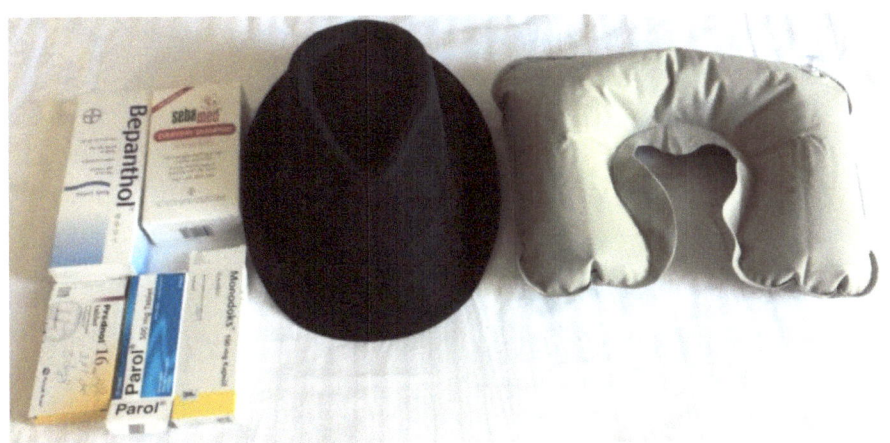

11.4. PROCEDURE SCOPE AND BASIC PARAMETERS

Type- Manual Follicular Unit Extraction (FUE)

Size- 4250 grafts transplanted

Scope- Hairline, top and crown area

Price of the procedure- 1800 Euro (about 2100 USD) based on the current exchange rate

Duration- approximately 6 hours in total - 1.5-2 hours for the extraction and about 3.5-4 hours for the actual transplanting + a 30 min lunch break.

Number of hair technicians involved in my procedure- 4

Level of pain and physical discomfort from 1 to 10(1 being the lowest)- 2. I was barely able to feel anything

Level of communication with the clinic and follow through - 8. Almost everyone involved - the clinic's coordinator, company driver, the chief surgeon and also owner of the clinic, and the four technicians simultaneously working on my head were quite fluent in English and friendly, so I didn't experience any significant language barrier.

Clinic's Location- Istanbul, Turkey

11.5.   INCLUSIONS IN THE PRICE OF THE PROCEDURE

Hotel accommodation (3 nights in a great hotel near the clinic)- I would give it a 9 since I was happy with the hotel, the room, and the level of service.

Transportation from and back to the airport and the clinic with a company(clinic) car and an English speaking designated driver

All necessary post-surgery medications and aftercare products- medical 5.5 PH shampoo, inflatable travel neck pillow (the one provided by the clinic turned out to be quite uncomfortable for sleeping so I was happy to have brought a special pillow), regular fedora hat

Post-surgery follow up and aftercare **by the clinic** - I'd give it a ten since they had a great follow up procedure in place and kept sending me regular follow up emails throughout the recuperation period.

11.6. PROCEDURE'S TIMELINE

8:30 am -   Hotel pick up by a clinic's designated driver

9:00 am -   Face-to-face meeting, and final go over with the head surgeon

9:30 am -   Hair trimming and hairline design by a designated specialist

10:00am-12 pm- Local anesthetic shots* and follicle extraction (manual via FUE technique)

12 pm- 12:45 pm - Lunch break (the clinic provided the lunch)

1pm-5:00 pm-   Transplanting stage

5:00-5:15 pm-   Bandage placement (on the donor area)**

6:00 pm -   Hotel drop off by the clinic's driver.

The next day

9:30 am -   Pick up by the clinic's driver and drop off at the clinic

10:00 am-   Donor area bandage removal

10:30 am-   Post-op aftercare instructions***

11:00 am-   Drop off back at the hotel

* The anesthetic shots usually last for a couple of days after the procedure, therefore I didn't experience any pain whatsoever. My surgeon provided me with the painkillers necessary to offset the physical discomfort after the hair transplant procedure.

** My donor area was wrapped with bandages and surgical absorbent pads, carefully placed onto my donor area to keep it sterile.

*** Final instructions on how to handle the first ten critical post days after the procedure.

12. PRE- AND POST-SURGERY PICTURES

Pre-op pics

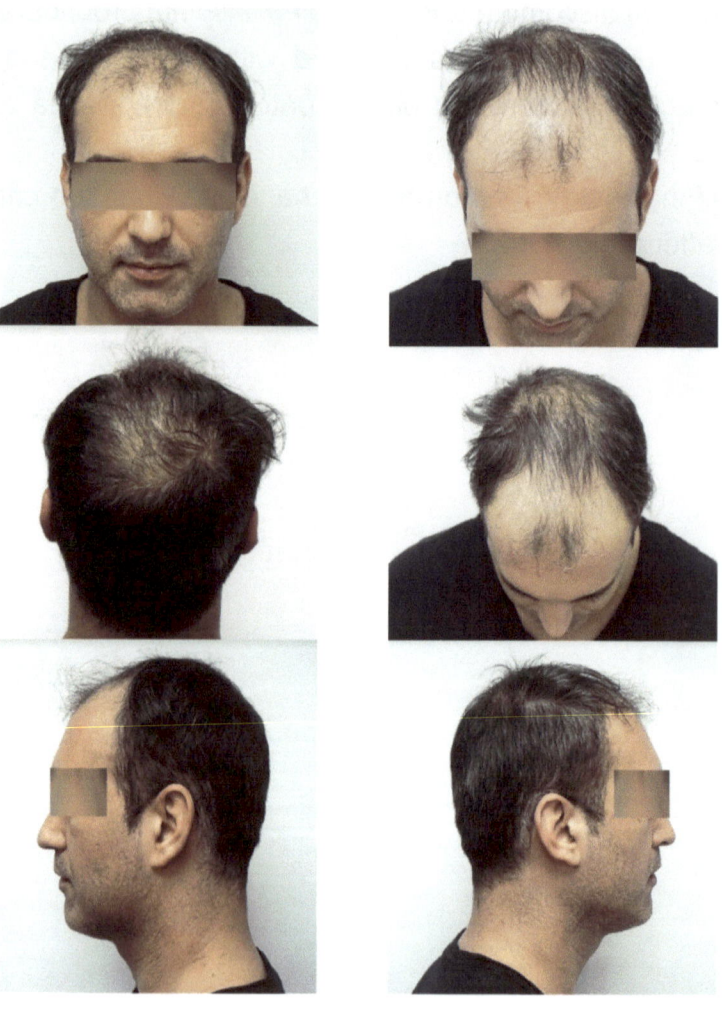

Post-surgery photos

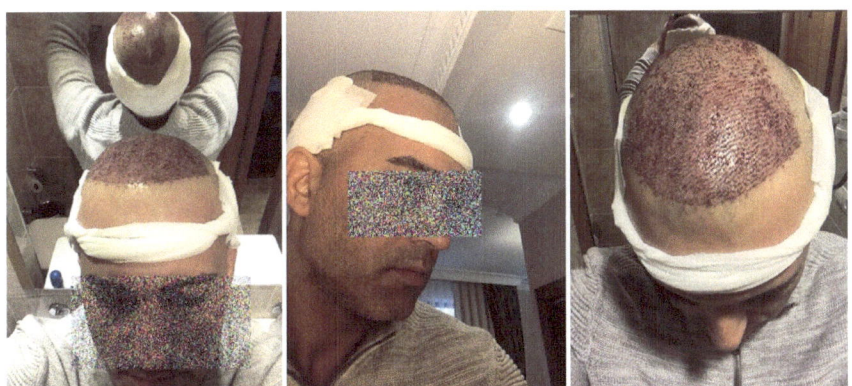

Day 1

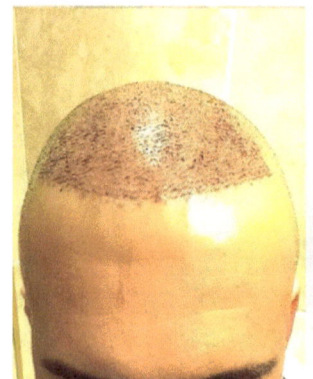 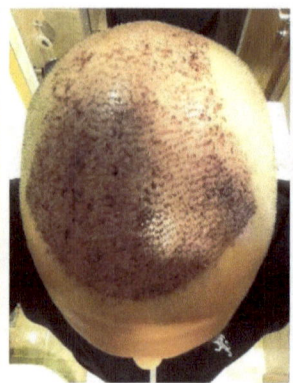 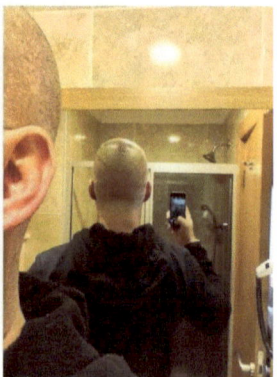

Day 2

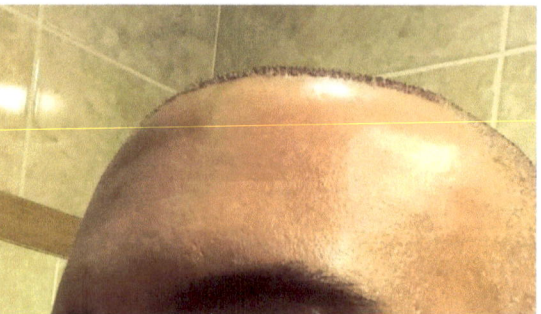

Head swelling

day 3

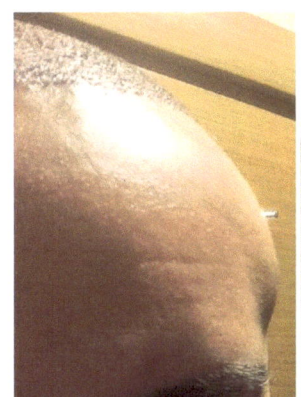 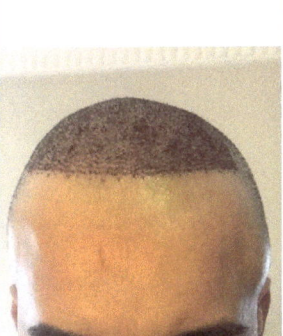 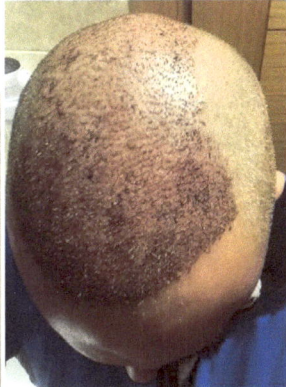

day 4

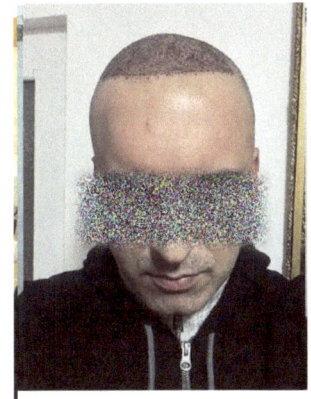 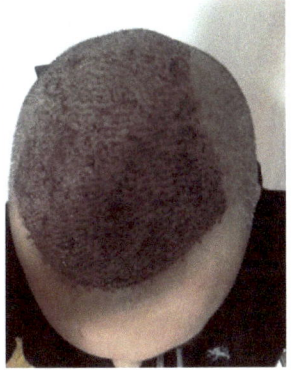 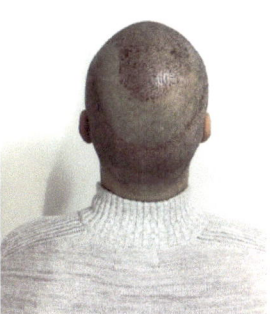

day 5

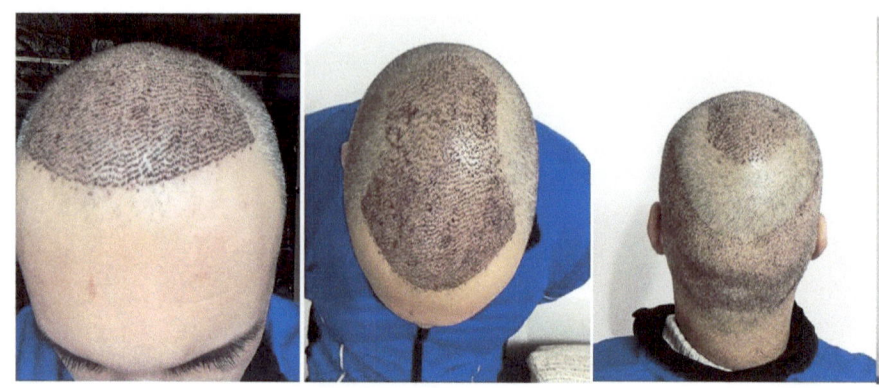

day 6

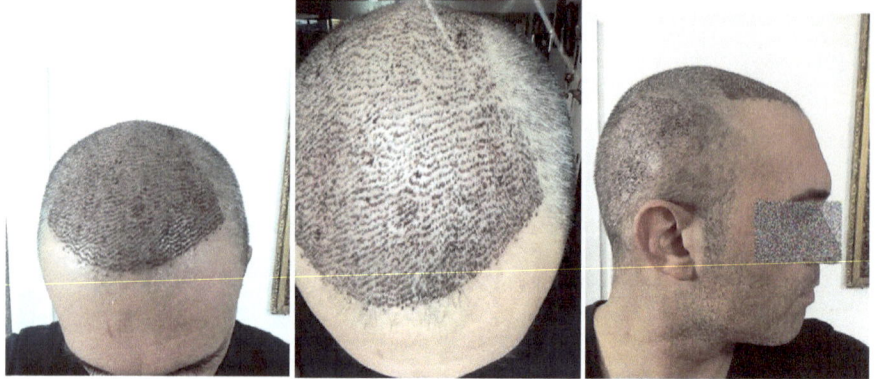

Day 7 - scratch

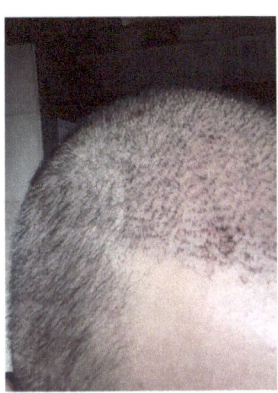 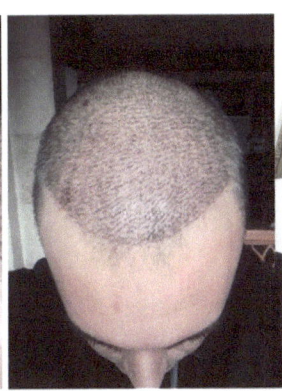 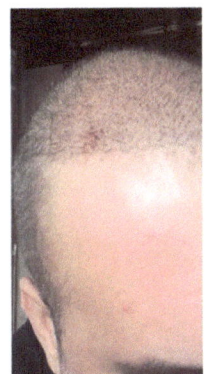

I scratched my head in my sleep on the 7th day and pulled out a few grafts.

In order to avoid the same happening to you use some sort of a head protector while you sleep or cut your

fingernails deep so you avoid causing damage to your newly transplanted hair follicles.

Day 10 -Immediate growth

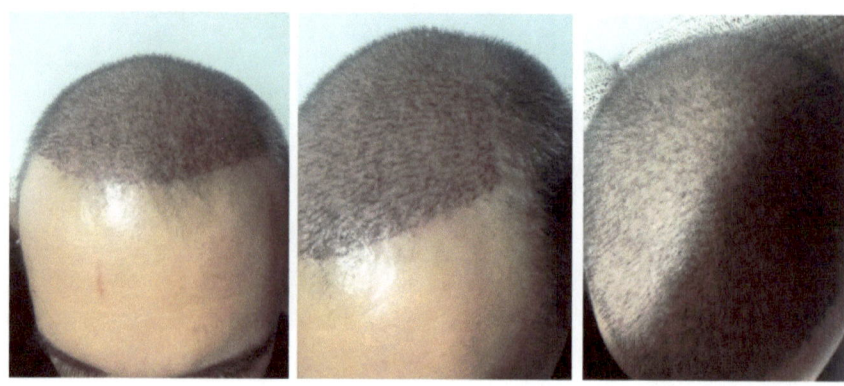

Day 20- Beginning of the "shock loss" stage

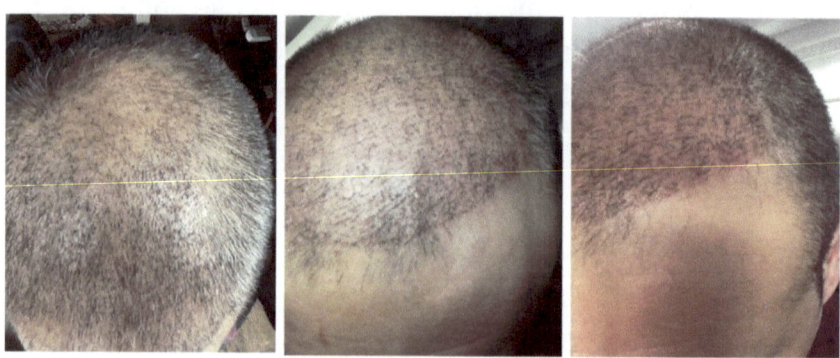

Day 45

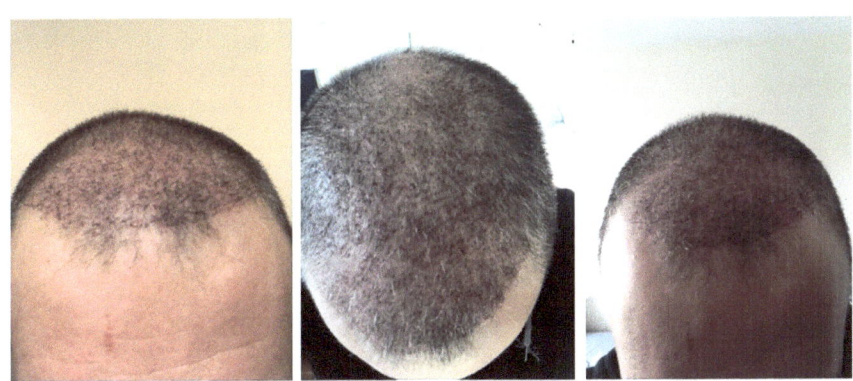

Day 70

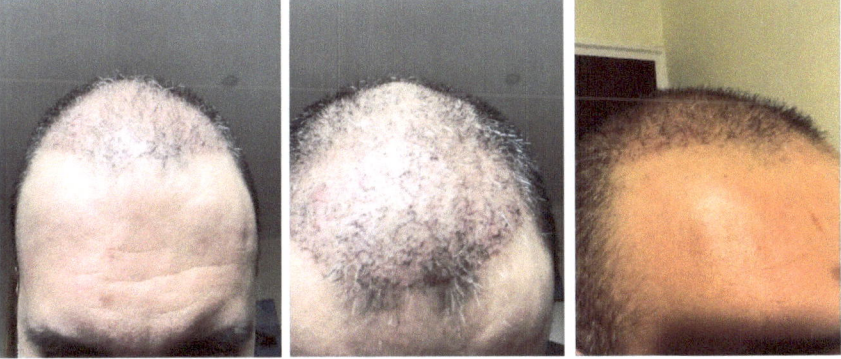

Day 95

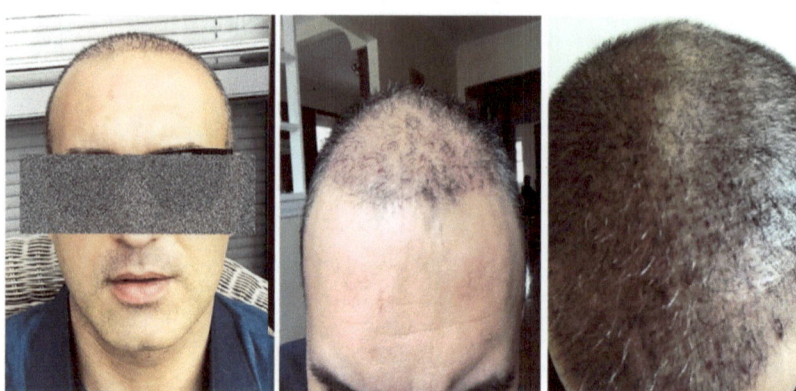

Good news!

The shock loss stage is officially over. The newly transplanted hair follicles have already started to produce new hairs, which naturally will take you to the so-called

"itchy stage" when your scalp will begin itching due to the new hairs breaking out through the epidermal layer of your scalp.

At this point, your transplanted follicles are deeply rooted, and you shouldn't be concerned about pulling them out. So it is ok to scratch.

However, try to do it gently, so you don't break the new hairs and slow down

the growth of your new hair.

Month 4

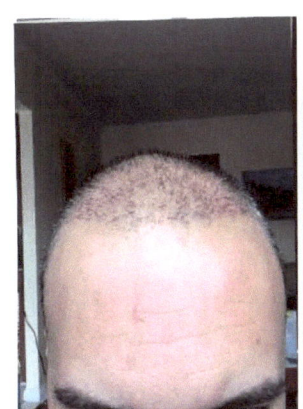 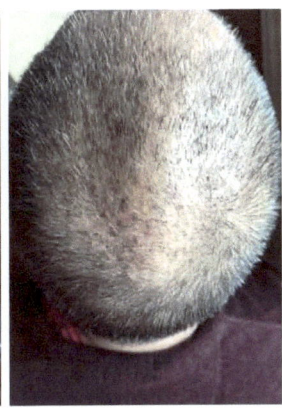 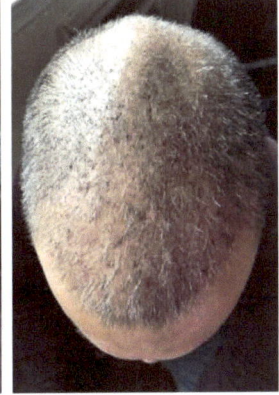

Month 5

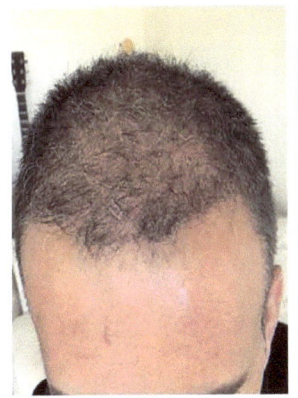 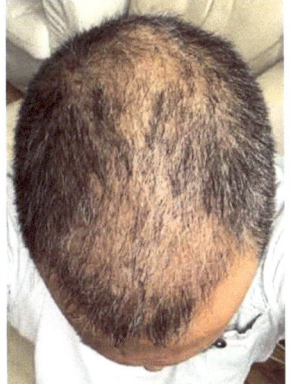 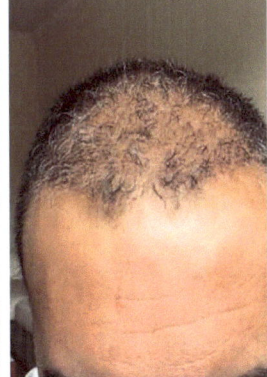

Month 6- massive growth

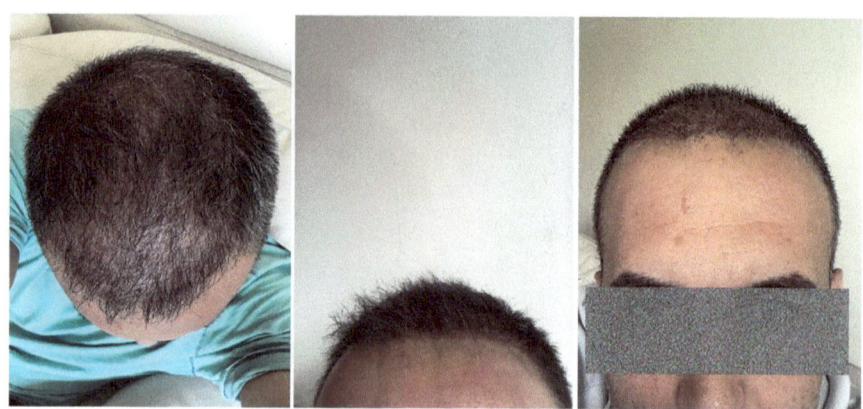

Month 7

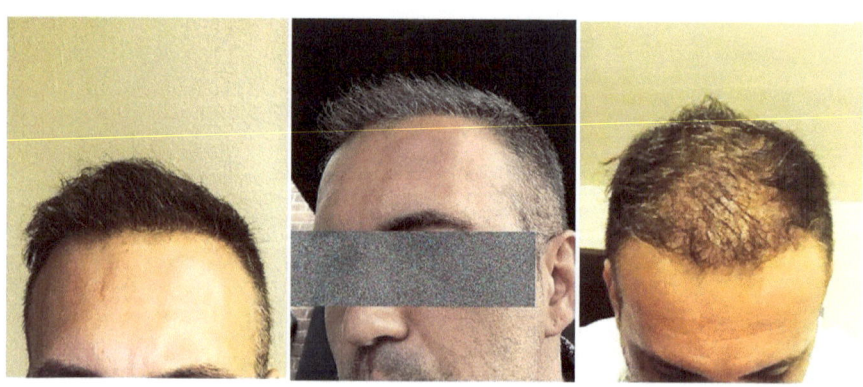

Month 8

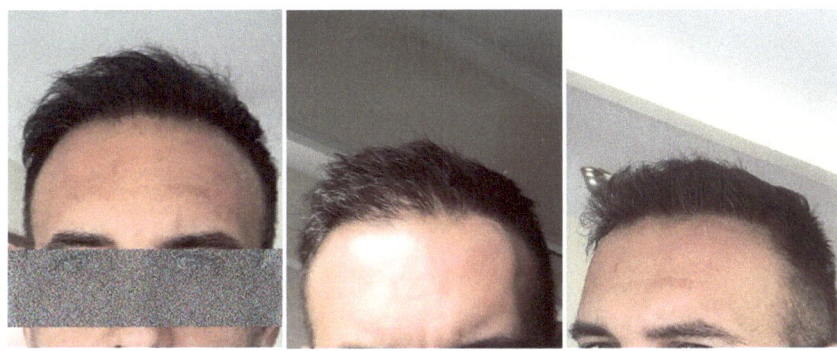

Month 9

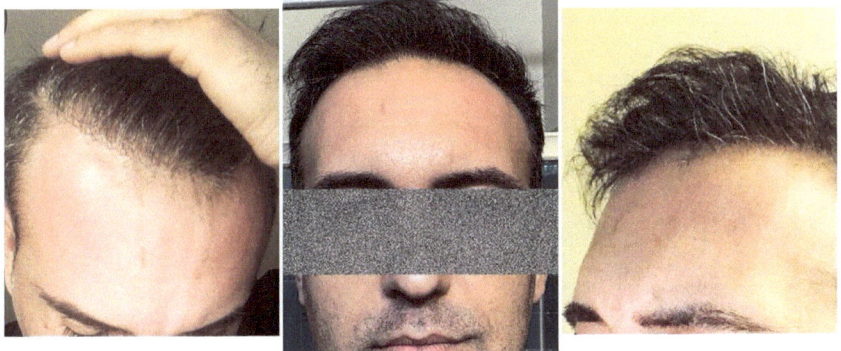

Month 12

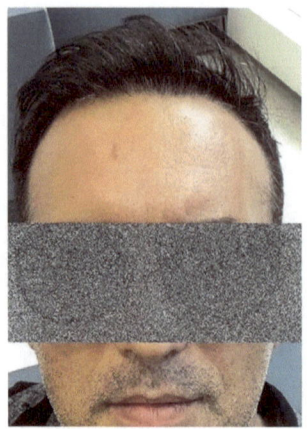
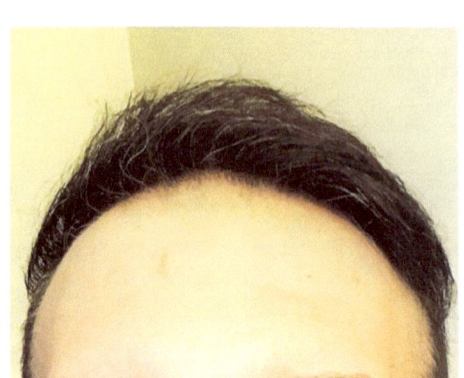

Month 18 - Final result

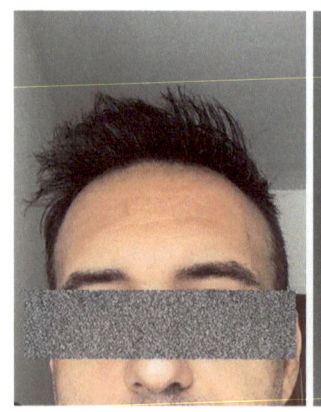
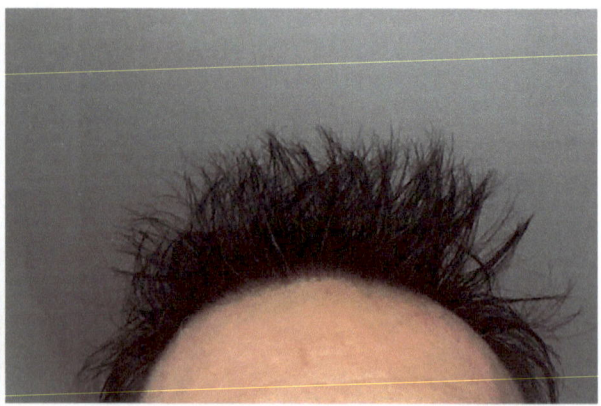

24 Months after the procedure

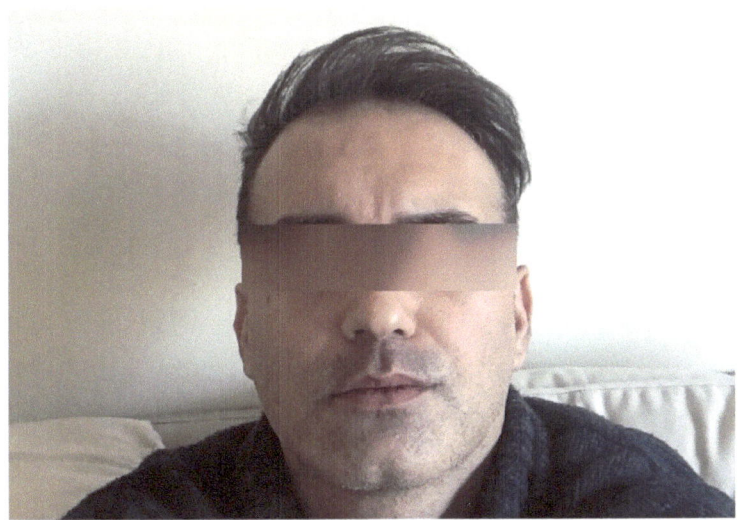

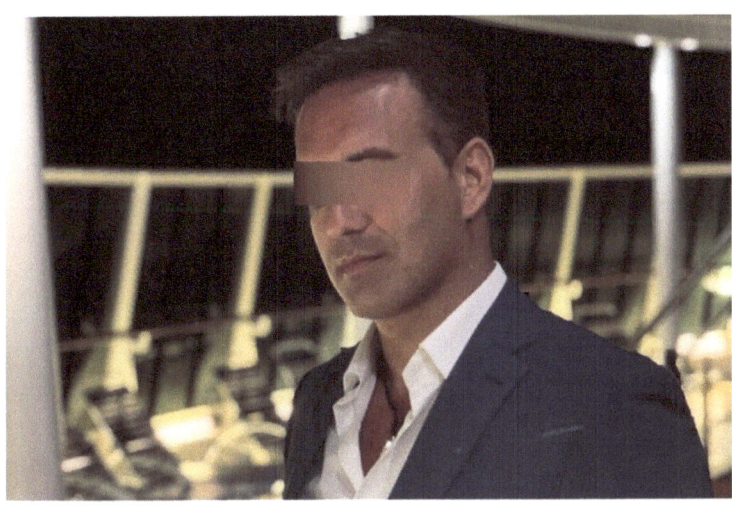

13. CONCLUSION. FINAL THOUGHTS AND RECOMMENDATIONS BY THE AUTHOR

Besides the hair follicles' genetic predisposition to the morbid impact of dihydrotestosterone, the health and look of our hair is also influenced by a variety of side factors – both internal (physiological and psychological) and external (environmental) ones.

Our general health condition, diet, exercising routine, stress levels, unhealthy habits and lifestyle in general, combined with the toxicity of the environment (worsened quality of food, water, and air) could also severely impact the health and look of our hair.

For me, the FUE hair transplant procedure turned out as desired and expected.

The post-op inconvenience was not as minor as described by the clinics, and in the hair forums so I ended up finding myself not as well prepared as I thought I would be.

Furthermore, it took a little longer than expected to be able to see tangible results.

I figured that it doesn't boil down to just getting the hair transplant done and that expediting the growth of the transplanted grafts involves continuous effort and dedication after the procedure.

The regular exercising, improved diet and cutting down on some unhealthy habits and routines didn't just help my hair re-grow much faster but also tangibly improved my general look, muscle tone, skin condition…, etc. I ended up getting all the positive side benefits of my continuous effort to achieve the maximum result from my hair transplant procedure. I would recommend a healthier lifestyle and routines to anyone looking to restore their hair completely.

I hope that this book will help you choose the right path in restoring your self-confidence and will help you to get prepared for your hair transplant procedure if that's the way you decide for yourselves.

STAY CONNECTED WITH THE AUTHOR.

Sign up on www.theMightyFollicle.com